Living a Positive Life in a Negative World

Living a Positive Life in a Negative World

My Uphill Journey

LINDA S. PLUNKETT, PhD

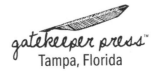

gatekeeper press™
Tampa, Florida

Living a Positive Life in a Negative World: My Uphill Journey

Published by Gatekeeper Press
7853 Gunn Hwy., Suite 209
Tampa, FL 33626
www.GatekeeperPress.com

Library of Congress Control Number: 2022952333

ISBN (paperback): 9781662928086
eISBN: 9781662928093

Dedication

I would like to dedicate this book to a dear friend, Mary Jane Peters (1938–2022), who passed away during the final stages of writing this book this past summer.

It was a difficult time, as she had been battling cancer for a number of years, and these past few months had become more and more challenging. Even then, Mary Jane was a "trooper," determined to continue her treatments, not wanting to give up the difficult fight.

She had expressed to me that she was so appreciative of the support of her loving family and friends.

Mary Jane was the mother of two, and a dear friend to so many people. She touched all of those around her with her tender love and compassion. Her positive attitude and strong faith in God were an inspiration to all. I feel so blessed personally to call her my friend.

I look forward to one day celebrating life with Mary Jane in a perfect place we call "heaven," where there will be no more pain and suffering, and where we will have unending joy!

Rest in peace, sweet Mary Jane. This book is dedicated to you.

Contents

SECTION TWO

SECTION THREE

Introduction

In October 2012, I heard the words I never expected to hear in a million years: "I'm sorry to tell you this, but you have a brain tumor." A nearly eight-hour brain surgery procedure followed. Afterwards, I felt mentally like an empty slate, with no thinking or problem-solving tools of any kind to successfully begin a new life. Recovery was extremely slow. I had to learn to walk again. I struggled with balance and had frequent falls around the house. In addition, I experienced anxiety and depression. I cried on a daily basis. I had throbbing headaches that encompassed the entire top of my head, the result of having my head cut open from ear to ear to remove the brain tumor. A much bigger issue, however, was my spiritual emptiness. I felt God had mysteriously left me, and this was my biggest dilemma of all. To heal, my brain surgeon told me that the "tennis ball-sized hole in my brain had to rewire itself," a phrase I didn't understand at the time. Hopelessness became my constant companion.

A few months later, gradual improvement was happening, but at a very slow pace. Thankfully, God was faithful in saving my life when I was literally at death's door, as chronicled in my previous book, *Supernatural Rescue*. I knew He was back in my life. However, I still seemed to have an inability to focus or problem-solve, and was miles away from being able to return help to other people via my beloved counseling practice. Then, more bad news came; after a day of testing at a major medical institution, I heard more difficult words. "I'm sorry to tell you this, but there's nothing we can do for you." I was in shock! *How could this be?* I asked myself. They were the most notable medical clinic in our area, and I had hopes they could provide massive solutions for my problems. All my hope was to no avail! At that point, I could have easily given up. But deep down inside of me, there was a voice of hope. At that moment in time, I truly believed that God, with His goodness, would not, could not, leave me in this horrible state of body, mind, and emotions.

I would like to tell you that at the conclusion of my first book, *Supernatural Rescue*, the medication I began taking for fibromyalgia continued to help my pain and sleep issues. Unfortunately it did not. Life became a more extreme test the next few years of what seemed to be an unending cycle of pain and sleeplessness which lasted not months but years.

By the end of 2016, many prayers were answered. Eventually, through doing much study, the many hours of time and research provided helpful solutions for further healing and restoration of my body physically. More hours of time and prayer also answered my own questions involving my inner emotional and spiritual battles. It is my hope that some of the answers chronicled in this book may also of great benefit to others as well.

This book is broken down into three sections. Section One includes your physical body, which primarily relates to your surrounding environment. Section Two covers the area sometimes called the "soul," and encompasses your mind, will, and emotions. The final section looks at your spiritual side, and involves your relationship with God. I will be sharing my own personal struggles, and answers I discovered in the long process of finding solutions for my own issues. That said, one warning I do want to give right away, and that you should keep in mind throughout this book, is that **if you have any doubts about your ability to perform physical activities, be sure to consult with your doctor first before beginning any new exercise regimen.**

Others have reminded me that even if they did not experience the same issues with their body, brain, emotional, or even spiritual lives, they also could use helpful suggestions to give them hope for a better life. It is my desire and prayer that this book will also help readers in discovering tools for a happier future. Please always understand that although we are all constantly dealing with negative scenarios in the world around us, there is a God who loves us and still promises us positive hope for the future, filled with possibilities. Whatever you may be going through, never give up. Tomorrow is another day, and your story is not finished yet!

SECTION ONE

CHAPTER 1

Exercise After Brain Surgery: The Value of Walking

Can you imagine a brain doctor telling you a few days after your brain surgery that you had to walk? This was my scenario in December 2012. I could barely stand, let alone balance my body to take forward steps, and my doctor was instructing me with the following demand: "You have to walk."

As I began that painful process, due to much pain and dizziness resulting from the nearly eight-hour surgery, my steps were very unstable, and as the result of trying to walk I had many unanticipated falls. The hard surface beneath me was unforgiving and left resulting "souvenirs" consisting of bumps and bruises on my body. My husband, Jim, was a real trooper. The main method I used to get any quality walking in my schedule was to lean into his shoulder, and he literally dragged me around the mall as we attempted to get in walking repetitions during the busy holiday season.

Why did the doctor require this activity so soon after brain surgery? As I later learned, walking not only benefits the body, but also the brain. My brain needed to re-wire itself, and exercise was hugely important in my brain's healing. Gradually, I reached the point where I was able to walk unassisted without having frequent falls. Now, years later I still continue to make an effort to walk regularly, as I find it not only helps my balance and coordination but also positively aids my mental performance.

While I was recently researching the benefits of walking, I found many other reasons it may be beneficial for you to walk. The first five items on this list were reported in June of this year by the *Harvard Health Letter* newsletter:

1. Walking counteracts the effects of weight-promoting genes. Harvard researchers looked at over 12,000 cases and discovered that among the study participants, for those who walked briskly for an hour a day, the effects of those genes were cut in half.
2. A pair of studies at the University of Exeter confirmed that walking curbs cravings and intake of sugary snacks.
3. An American Cancer Society study found that walking an hour a day lowered the risk of developing breast cancer by 14%.
4. Walking eases joint pain. Several studies have confirmed that walking 5–6 miles a week may

prevent arthritis. Walking protects the joints, especially the knees and hips, by lubricating and strengthening the muscles that support them.

5. Walking boosts the immune function. A study of over 1,000 men and women found that those who walked at least twenty minutes five days a week had 43% fewer sick days than those who only exercised once a week. When they did get sick, it was for a shorter duration, and their symptoms were milder.

6. Additionally, Healthline.com states walking thirty minutes a day, five days a week can reduce your risk for heart disease by 19%. And your risk may reduce even more when you increase the duration or distance you walk per day.

7. Healthline.com also states walking may increase your energy level, increasing oxygen flow through the body as well as increasing hormones that increase energy levels, such as cortisol, epinephrine, and norepinephrine.

8. They also confirm that walking can improve your mood and your mental health. Studies show it can reduce anxiety, depression, and a negative mood. It can also boost self-esteem and reduce symptoms of social withdrawal. Aim for thirty minutes of brisk walking three days a week.

9. Healthline also states that walking can extend your life, as researchers have found that walking at an average pace compared to a slow pace resulted in a 20% reduced risk of overall death. But walking at a brisk or a fast pace of at least four miles an hour reduces the risk by 24%. The study looked at the association between walking at a faster pace and factors like overall causes of death, cardiovascular disease, and death from cancer.

10. It was also noted by Healthline that walking may promote clarity in thinking. A study that included four experiments compared people trying to think of new ideas while sitting or walking. Researchers discovered those participants did better while walking, particularly while walking outdoors.

So, don't be surprised at your next checkup if your doctor hands you a prescription to walk!

CHAPTER 2

Overweight and Unhappy: Time for "Upping my Game"

I was regularly walking, and for the most part improving my balance and getting my energy back. However, I still had considerable weight to lose. Taking steroids before and after brain surgery had caused sugar cravings, and I had put on considerable weight—over forty pounds, to be exact. Every time I looked in the mirror, I seemed to feel worse about myself. I remember feeling irritated with my husband Jim when he allowed someone to take a picture of us. I hated my overweight, out-of-shape appearance. I definitely needed to do something. In trying to do things to improve my brain performance and balance, I had neglected my overall physical conditioning. My body definitely showed the negative results. It was definitely time to "up my game" and make changes.

My son Brian, a personal trainer, encouraged me to return to the gym and get into a program of strength training. He has seen many people benefit from strength training and get back in shape. This was definitely the most out of shape I had ever been, weighing close to 200 pounds.

With making the time and putting forward effort to go to the gym two to three times a week, I began to see changes in my body. At sixty years of age, I felt my metabolism had slowed down, but thankfully the effort paid off and I gradually began to lose weight and firm up. I eventually dropped about three clothing sizes.

If you have never thought about weight training or strength training, I want to encourage you to at least consider it. During the past few years, more and more studies have shown that sensible strength training produces many health and fitness benefits. Key researchers have provided a wealth of data on the positive physiological responses to basic programs of strength exercise. Consider these twelve reasons to start to do strength training, originally found at ExerciseCoach.com:

1. Avoid muscle loss. According to an article in *Forbes*, the average adult loses 5–7 pounds of muscle mass per decade. Only strength exercise maintains our muscle mass and strength throughout our midlife years.
2. Avoid metabolic rate reduction. Strength training on a regular basis prevents the accompanying decrease in resting metabolic rate.

3. Increase muscle mass. Because most adults do not perform strength exercises, they need to first replace the muscle tissue that has been lost through inactivity. Twenty-five minutes of strength exercise three times a week would be the typically recommended program for men and women.

4. Increase metabolic rate. Adults who replace muscle through sensible strength exercise use more calories all day long, thereby reducing the likelihood of fat accumulation.

5. Reduce body fat. A 1994 study by nutritionist W.W. Campbell showed that strength training exercise produces four pounds of fat loss after three months of training, even though the subjects were eating 15% more calories per day.

6. Increase bone mineral density. The same training was shown in another study (Menkes 1993) to lead to increases in osteoproteins and mineral content.

7. Improve glucose metabolism.

8. Increase gastrointestinal transit time, which has been shown to lower colon cancer rate.

9. Reduce resting blood pressure.

10. Improve blood lipid levels.

11. Reduce lower back pain.

12. Reduce arthritis pain.

From my personal point of view, a consistent program of personal strength training allowed me to not only feel better and improve my level of physical fitness, but ultimately aided in improving my personal self-confidence, as I continued to lose weight and fit into smaller sizes. Best wishes as you pursue your own regimen to gain a stronger and healthier body.

CHAPTER 3

"Empty Head Dilemma:" Best Practices for Brain Improvement

As I briefly mentioned in the introduction, after the large tumor was removed during brain surgery, I was told my brain had to re-wire itself. I didn't understand the concept at the time.

The term "neuroplasticity" or brain plasticity simply means that our brains are constantly changing. Just as my brain needed to re-wire an empty space, all of our brains possess the remarkable ability to reorganize pathways, create new connections, and in some cases, even create new neurons throughout your entire lifetime. Your brain changes and adapts in response to experience. This is great news for people such as myself, who have had brain injury or a serious surgery that has severely affected their brains. However, the news is also significant for those who may be beginning to experience the effects of brain aging.

We now know that for good brain health, we need both physical and mental exercise. Recent studies have shown that physical exercise is as important as mental exercise when it comes to keeping your brain fit. A number of studies show that exercise can promote growth of new brain cells, enlarge the memory center, improve IQ scores, and help prevent brain deterioration as you age.

When I first came home after brain surgery, I only had the ability to sit at the dining room table and put together a few traditional table puzzles. Then eventually, I graduated to trying to do more difficult crossword and sudoku puzzles. As I also increased my walking and added strength training, I believe all of these activities greatly helped my brain improvement. Physical exercise in particular prompts nerve cells to release a growth factor called brain-derived neurotrophic factor, or BDNF. BDNF triggers numerous other chemicals that promote neural health and directly benefit cognitive functions including learning.

According to the *Harvard Health Letter* newsletter, physical exercise helps memory and thinking through both direct and indirect means. The benefits of exercise come directly from its ability to reduce insulin resistance, reduce inflammation, and simulate the release of the growth factors. These growth factors affect the health of the brain cells and the growth of new blood vessels in the brain, and even the abundance and survival of these new brain cells. Many studies have suggested that the parts of the brain that control thinking and memory, the prefrontal frontal cortex and the medial temporal cortex, have a greater volume in people who exercise versus people who don't. Even more exciting is the finding that engaging in a program of regular exercise of moderate intensity over six months to a year is associated with an increase in volume of selected brain regions, according to Dr. Scott McGuinness of Harvard Medical School. In addition, a study chronicled in the *Journal of Alzheimer's Disease* by Dr. Ozioma Okonkwo of the University of Wisconsin School of Medicine states that exercise might be a simple way for people to cut down their risk for memory loss and Alzheimer's disease, even for those who are genetically at risk for the disease.

Dr. Okonkwo's research has also shown that exercise can diminish the impact of brain changes and cognition, not just prevent it. "Exercise is the full package," he says. He adds that exercise likely improves brain health through a variety of ways. It makes the heart beat faster, which increases blood flow to the brain. The blood delivers oxygen, which is a good thing since the brain is the biggest consumer of oxygen in the body, as we discussed previously. It also increases BDNF, which helps repair and protect brain cells from degeneration as well as help new brain cells and neurons.

So, what are the best exercises for the brain? There are a variety of opinions. In general, doctors agree that the best types of exercise are those that help increase the heart rate, affecting the heart health of the individual in a positive way. Those types of exercises may include aerobic walking, weight training (and especially interval training), and even dancing. Whatever you choose, remember that if the activity is new for you, your body needs time to adjust to the new activity.

After I began working on my own exercise program, even with regular walking and going to the gym for a number of months, I still continued to have struggles with balance and coordination. To combat this, I made an attempt to return to an activity that I dearly loved before my brain surgery. That activity was ballroom dancing. I had not danced for a period time, but I soon found that dancing was not only great exercise for my body physically, but really seemed to improve my struggling brain in the process. I returned to taking lessons with my former instructor Chris, and found the challenges involved with regaining the old memory of steps I had formerly learned invigorating. Learning new choreography resulted in major positive changes.

An article published by Stanford University states that not only does dancing benefit our health in a physical way, but also provides stress reduction and increased serotonin levels, with an accompanying sense of well-being. The article goes further to say that "frequent dancing apparently makes us smarter." The major study adds to the growing evidence that stimulating one's mind by dancing can ward off Alzheimer's disease and other dementia, much as physical exercise can keep a body fit.

You may have heard of a *New England Journal of Medicine* study on the effects of recreational activities on mental acuity in aging. They studied activities such as reading, writing for pleasure, doing puzzles, playing cards, and playing musical instruments. In addition, they looked at physical activities such as tennis, golf, swimming, biking, dancing, walking, and doing housework. The focus was the mind, and the results indicated that almost none of the physical exercises appeared to offer any protection against dementia. There was only one exception. The only physical activity to offer protection against dementia was frequent dancing. Below lists some of their findings:

- Reading: 35% reduced risk of dementia
- Bicycling and swimming: 0%
- Doing crosswords at least four days a week: 47%
- Playing golf: 0%

- Dancing frequently: 76%. This activity was the greatest risk reduction of any activity studied, cognitive or physical.

Why was this the case? There are many examples over the decades that have shown we increase our mental capacity by exercising our cognitive process. The essence of intelligence is making decisions. The best advice in improving your mental acuity is to involve yourself in activities that require split-second, rapid-fire decision-making, as opposed to rote memory, doing the same things over and over. Dancing integrates several brain functions at once—kinesthetic, rational, musical, and emotional—further increasing your neural connectivity.

Remember earlier when we discussed neuroplasticity? One way to grow your brain and create new pathways is to do something new; not just dancing, but anything new. Take a class to challenge your mind. This will help you develop new pathways in your brain. According to brain plasticity expert Dr. Michael Merzenich, engaging in new activities throughout your life, staying socially active, and practicing "mindfulness" are other ways to boost brain function.

Take time to challenge yourself to try something new. Tomorrow is a new day . . . to enjoy better brain health!

CHAPTER 4

Eating For a Better Brain

After brain surgery, I was at such an extremely low point, physically and mentally. I realized that the empty hole in my head was the cause of so many problems. I was told literally that there was no way to determine how the re-wiring would take place or what outcome to expect. In the past, prior to the brain surgery, I felt I ate reasonably healthy. But honestly, until 2012, I don't recall that I had any major medical issues that concerned me. Now, at an all-time low, I felt the urgency to change everything!

I was curious, as I researched the best foods for brain health, if anything had changed since I explored the same research seven years ago. After researching several top sources for boosting brain function and memory, I found very few changes. Before I list these, I want to be emphatic about the fact you need to choose your foods wisely. Consult your doctor before making rash decisions, to be sure you don't have food allergies or interactions with your current medications. For example, two of the foods I am going to list that are recommended for good brain health I personally cannot consume due to food allergies, so I have had to find substitutes that provide similar nutritional benefits.

The following are the top foods several sources list in order boost brain function:

1. Fatty or oily fish are good sources for omega-3s, which help in building membranes around each cell in the body, including the brain. Omega-3s play a role in sharpening memory and improving mood, as well as protecting your brain against cognitive decline (MedicalNewsToday.com). These fish may include salmon, herring, trout, albacore tuna, and sardines.

2. Broccoli is packed with antioxidants. It is also very high in vitamin K, a fat-soluble vitamin that is essential for forming sphingolipids, a type of fat that is densely packed into brain cells. In addition, broccoli contains vitamin C and flavonoids, and these antioxidants can further boost a person's brain health. In addition to broccoli, kale and leafy greens also contain similar key ingredients (MedicalNewsToday.com).

3. Eggs are a very good source of vitamins B6 and B12, as well as folic acid. Recent research suggests these vitamins may prevent brain shrinkage and delay cognitive decline. Choline

found in eggs is also shown to benefit the brain (MedicalNewsToday.com).

4. Coffee contains caffeine and antioxidants that can support brain health. Included in the positive effects include increased alertness, improved mood, and sharpened concentration. The only reported downside reported by some people is inability to sleep. Coffee is not doctor-recommended for all people.

5. Berries contain flavonoid antioxidants which help reduce inflammation and oxidative stress. A 2014 study notes that the antioxidant compounds on berries have many positive effects on the brain including improved communication between brain cells, reduced inflammation throughout the body, increased plasticity, which helps brain cells form new connections, boosting learning and memory, and reduced or delayed age-related neurodegenerative disease and cognitive decline. Berries that can boost brain health include strawberries, blackberries, blueberries, black currants, and mulberries (MedicalNewsToday.com).

6. Nuts and seeds are likely good for the brain because of their omega-3 fatty acids and antioxidants. In particular, vitamin E protects

cells from oxidative stress caused by free radicals. This may be particularly helpful as a person ages. The nuts and seeds with the highest amounts of vitamin K include sunflower seeds, almonds, and hazelnuts (MedicalNewsToday.com).

7. Dark chocolate and cocoa powder are packed with brain boosting compounds, including flavonoids, caffeine, and antioxidants. The flavonoids in chocolate gather in the areas of the brain that deal with learning and memory. Researchers believe that these compounds may enhance memory and also help slow down age-related mental decline (Healthline.com).

The bottom line is that many foods can keep your brain healthy. Some may possibly also improve memory and concentration. Some may go further to reduce the risk of stroke and age-related diseases, such as Parkinson's or Alzheimer's. Brain boosting foods tend to contain one or more of the following (MedicalNewsToday.com):

1. Antioxidants such as flavonoids or vitamin E
2. B vitamins
3. Healthy fats
4. Omega fatty acids

Beyond including some of these top foods in your diet, I highly recommend seeing your medical professional to determine which changes to your current diet may be healthy for you. Also, it's always a great idea to discover, through your current lab tests, any particular deficiencies that may exist in your particular body, and how to best address these situations. For me personally, I have found that annual, and in some cases, semi-annual testing offers huge benefits, in terms of making changes for a healthier future.

I also want to mention in this section that additional supplements, as recommended by your doctor or nutritionist, may help you meet your personal goals. Not all major medical institutions seem to agree on the value of brain supplements. That is a matter of opinion. In my personal situation, that of recovering from brain surgery and trying to manage fibromyalgia, in which I have had many unique issues, I believe all of these have been improved by taking supplements. As my physician's office added supplements to my daily routine, my sleep in particular has improved. I also have felt some improvement by expanding my vitamin supplement routine to include nootropics to help me boost my cognitive functions. As I previously mentioned, there seems to be a big difference of opinion between "experts" in this field of research. I recommend seeing your medical professional to determine if adding any new supplements is the right course of action for you.

Most importantly, make healthy eating your first priority. Your body and brain will thank you for it!

CHAPTER 5

Worse than Brain Surgery Recovery: My Battle with "Fibromyalgia"

I am reluctant to use the term "fibromyalgia," even nearly ten years after I received that diagnosis, which is why I put it in quotation marks in the chapter's title. There is still so much confusion and conflicting opinions regarding the meaning of this term. Even today, in autumn 2022, as I Google articles there is huge disagreement as to its definition, origin of symptoms, and treatment. WebMD states that fibromyalgia is thought to be the result of overactive nerves which can last for years. Although, again, there is no consensus to the cause, WebMD suggests that the lowered pain thresholds may be caused by a reduced effectiveness of the body's natural endorphin painkillers, and there can be an ongoing cycle of pain and fatigue. The doctor who diagnosed my condition commented that my case was "classic," due to my experience of having to go through a nearly eight-hour brain surgery. He also stated it is frequently caused by any major trauma to the brain.

I am going to tell you my story dealing with fibromyalgia, which may be very different from yours. However, it is my hope that through my struggle to understand my own body and find solutions, some of them in unexpected ways, you might find hope for yourself or someone else who is struggling with chronic pain and sleep cycles.

It all started for me back in 2013, about eight and a half months after I had brain surgery and a large tumor had been removed from my frontal brain lobe. Let me quote a paragraph from my previous book, *Supernatural Rescue*:

I awoke one morning on a seemingly normal day. The sun was shining. The birds were singing. But my physical body was telling me that this day is anything but normal. I suddenly realized that I had chronic pain across my hips and shoulders. The thought crossed my mind, Maybe I slept in the wrong position?

I will get a better night's sleep tonight and tomorrow it will all be better. Regrettably, the following night's sleep was not the solution. The pain in my shoulders and hips caused me to toss and turn all night long. No matter what position I chose, there was pain, and the pain kept me awake. I tried various over-the-counter pain and sleep aids, but nothing seemed to help. What was happening? And then additional pains manifested themselves. My elbows started hurting and I could feel pain in my jaw area. What on earth is happening? Is my body gradually deteriorating from head to toe?

Because of the new pain, I saw the dentist that week, but to no avail. I had no dental issues affecting my jaw area. My body continued to ache, and I continued to have chronic pain, losing many hours of sleep. I began to feel like a zombie. I was behaving badly, irritable and short-tempered from lack of sleep. I am embarrassed to say it, but I began to hate myself for my bad behavior. One person close to me also considered my problems could be psychosomatic, or "all in my head." This was also embarrassing because I had earned a PhD in Biblical Psychology and had a practice helping people for fifteen years. And yet here I was, in my own words, "a total mess."

The only thing I could possibly think could be the cause of the physical pain problem was arthritis. I was thinking I might be in the early stages of rheumatoid arthritis or osteoarthritis, as previous to the brain surgery, I had experienced occasional pain in my hands. At that time, I had just taken an over-the-counter pain medication. Unfortunately, it took a couple of weeks to see a rheumatologist, and then there was another wait to get the results from the blood work. When I finally returned on the follow-up visit, I was hopeful that with the correct diagnosis and prescription drug, maybe I could have less pain and be able to sleep again.

The doctor was a specialist at a well-known clinic in the area, but I was in no way prepared for the news he was about to give me, that there was no indication of any arthritis in my body, other than very minor osteoarthritis in my hands. My hands were not the issue; pretty much everywhere else in my body was the issue. I asked him, "So to what do you attribute this widespread pain?" His answer shocked me—fibromyalgia. He explained that I had experienced a major trauma to my brain as a result of going through a nearly eight-hour brain surgery. He handed me an article about the condition and a pain prescription with some added advice: "If you go to go bed and get up at the same time every day, I'm sure you'll be fine." I personally felt his assessment was a gross oversimplification of my new "condition." The pain prescription did not work. Neither did the following one, nor the prescriptions to help me sleep. I began to feel seriously disorientated due to lack of sleep.

Unfortunately, my situation got worse. A month later when I was descending the stairs in my home, it was like a bad "blast from the past." I mentally thought I was at the bottom of the stairs, when in fact I was not. I missed five steps and went spiraling downward. I had experienced similar falls when I was struggling to walk again after brain surgery. But this time, when I hit the tile at the bottom of the stairs, I heard a popping sound. I had broken my ankle. All I could think of was, all those months doing balance therapy, to learn how to effectively walk again, and now this happens!

Now on crutches, I was again confined to the main floor. I hobbled across the family room and dining room to the half-bath at the end of the hall, and just like former days, the couch became my permanent bed. At this point, I was still somewhat overweight and I found using crutches painful, as I wasn't used to having to support my entire body with my arms. Walking was difficult. A few weeks later, the doctor prescribed a walking boot and physical therapy to strengthen the injured ankle. After a few weeks of rehabilitation, I graduated to tennis shoes, which I gladly celebrated.

I started to question if maybe there was a chance my brain tumor had returned. I had previously been warned that the type of tumor I had previously might return. With the pain and sleep issues still continuing, and with my latest falling incident leaving me in a quandary, I decided the best course of action was to have another MRI. Thankfully, no panic attack this time in the MRI machine, and good news from the doctor: no new brain tumor. When I questioned him regarding my fall, he answered, "It was from the effects of your fibromyalgia."

Although the next couple of years were very difficult, somehow I managed to get by with my faith and my supportive family. I was able to return to part-time counseling again. In my weakness, God used me to personally help a couple of other people who were in a worse condition. One thing I've learned is that as bad as you might feel, there is always someone whose condition is worse. It makes you feel grateful for the blessings you may still be able to celebrate, in spite of your condition. I also learned to look at my cup as half-full instead of half-empty, to still be able to give thanks to God for the small things in life. Also, I am thankful to him for allowing happy outcomes to come out of bad situations. You can read more of this period of time, and what I learned from my experiences, in my previous book, *Supernatural Rescue*.

Although at the end of the book, in 2015, I was taking an expensive prescription drug that I thought was my "miracle drug," which finally allowed me to sleep regularly eight hours and awake without pain, I am sad to tell you that the effects were unfortunately not permanent. However, in the following two chapters, it is my desire to share with you more information regarding what I have learned that greatly improved my fibromyalgia. I believe it is probably true when some articles say that there is not a proven cure for fibromyalgia. Having said that, I do believe in miracles. Meanwhile, whatever you are going through currently, I want to urge you to never give up! There are times I wanted to give up, but thankfully I did not.

Today, some people have describe me as a walking miracle. Ephesians tells us that we have a God "who can do immeasurably more than we ask or imagine." My life is evidence of this fact.

CHAPTER 6

An Unexpected Breakthrough

As I reported at the end of the last chapter, unfortunately the great results from the prescription medication I took to remedy the fibromyalgia pain and sleep issues did not last. It was nice while it lasted, but less than approximately four months later, I was back to square one. I did my very best to press forward in spite of the pain and lack of sleep, refusing to give up, even though life continued to be quite difficult. The future was unknown, but I still hadn't given up hope that God would provide me a more permanent solution.

One of the activities I attempted to continue to participate in was ballroom dancing, in spite of feeling at times somewhat unbalanced and even experiencing occasional dizziness. Having said that, I felt the challenge of trying to constantly learn new dance steps and take lessons with a pro dance teacher vastly helped my balance and coordination, as well as my brain.

In early 2016, my husband Jim and I decided to attend a ballroom dance competition on one of the largest ships in the world. At that point in time, I had been struggling with the pain and sleep issues, only experiencing very temporary relief from fibromyalgia, for over two and a half years. But at some point in time, my mindset began to change. I made the decision to stop limiting myself. I created a new habit of doing activities in spite of not getting a good night's sleep. This was probably was not the greatest decision I ever made, and you will soon understand why. I was pushing myself because, quite frankly, I didn't want to give up living life to its fullest or miss out on activities I really enjoyed any longer. At that time, I made the decision to adopt as my motto "fake it 'til you make it."

It was a large cruise ship, so after dancing multiple heats in the ballroom, and then having to make the long walk back to my cabin on the other side of the ship, one night I found myself particularly fatigued and exhausted. As I recall, the prior night I did not get any sleep at all—zero sleep. It was not the first day on the ship, and we had already competed a couple of times. So, long story short, as I struggled physically to walk back to my room after a very long day, my knee totally collapsed, and I limped back to the cabin in excruciating pain. I was so disappointed not to be able complete the dance competition. However, my biggest issue was not that; it was just having the ability to walk. With my husband's help, I managed to get to the medical clinic. A large supportive compression boot allowed me to manage to maneuver, at least until I got back home to have an X-ray to determine further treatment.

My meniscal tears were the result of overuse, overdoing an activity without proper rest, but possibly also the results of early osteoarthritis. My body was also showing evidence of this in that my finger joints were also looking swollen. Upon consulting with my foundational medicine physician, he highly recommended an IV of mesenchymal stem cells for my knee injury. He said he personally had used them when he had major knee issues. He told me that had had had similar tears and osteoarthritis, and that his knee had been bone on bone. He said in a relatively short time, his knee was transformed. As I wanted to have full healing and also not have to go down the path of having surgery, I determined this to be the right course of action.

It was explained to me that these stem cells were derived from umbilical cords from afterbirth and the miracle was that these stem cells are "specialized cells that know what you need and where you need it, and they go there and become it." While mesenchymal stem cells are known to repair muscle, bone cartilage, and tendons, what happened after my stem cell treatment was completely unexpected. Not only did my knee totally heal, and no surgery was needed, but the stem cells provided an even greater and more miraculous result. The stem cells greatly reduced my fibromyalgia.

It was reduced to the point that pain was much less frequent, and that for the first time in a long time I started to have more frequent nights when I was able to fall asleep in a reasonable time and awaken well-rested. What a great personal victory, which greatly changed my life for the positive. It was definitely a game changer. I am so grateful to God for this unexpected blessing.

A new study posted on Nature.com in 2022 by the International Society for Cell and Gene Therapy provides an update on the recent clinical applications for the treatment of many human diseases, one of them being neurological disorders. This may potentially be exciting news for people who have not been able to find a treatment that works for them. I highly recommend reading this research to see if stem cells have been used to treat your particular condition. If so, you may want to consider a medical consultation.

In addition to the being treated with stem cells, I discovered other research which I have also found to help in better managing my remaining pain and sleep issues. As I was reminded, there is not a single "cure" for fibromyalgia. Although the stem cells helped immensely, there were still more changes I could make to live a healthier life. These I will share with you in the following chapter.

If you are still experiencing medical issues involving your body and or brain, don't give up. Sometimes it can be helpful to read articles online and seek different opinions from researchers and practitioners. The great news is that new studies are being conducted all the time. Tomorrow is a new day, filled with possibilities for a better future.

CHAPTER 7

Going the Distance: Finding New Strategies for a Better Body and Brain

As I mentioned in the last chapter, it was great to have the great improvement for my fibromyalgia after being treated with stem cells for my knee injury on the cruise ship. As a result, I now was able to have less sleepless nights and less pain, which was a great news! However, I continued to seek additional help to stabilize or even lower the number of the bad days, in which didn't get enough quality rest and as a result suffered pain the following day. In this section, I am going to share a few strategies that worked for me.

Eating for Less Pain

One of the first big discoveries I made was when I discovered my pain was in part the result of inflammation. Inflammation is defined by WebMD as "a process by which your body's white blood cells and the things they make protect you from infection from outside invaders, such as bacteria and viruses." But in some diseases, like arthritis, your immune system triggers inflammation when there are no invaders to fight off. In these autoimmune diseases, your immune system acts as if regular tissues are infected or somehow unusual, causing damage. Inflammation can be either short-lived (acute) or long-lasting (chronic). Acute inflammation goes away in within hour or days. Chronic inflammation can last months or years, even after the first trigger is gone. Conditions linked to chronic inflammation include cancer, heart disease, diabetes, and Alzheimer's disease. Also, other conditions that may be linked to inflammation include many types of arthritis, fibromyalgia, and lower neck and back pain. Some of the symptoms of inflammation may include redness, pain and stiffness, Additionally, inflammation may also cause flu-like symptoms including fever, chills, and headaches.

For me personally, it was a huge revelation that I could battle my inflammation by adopting an anti-inflammatory diet. Although I haven't always followed the diet exclusively, I've seen an overall decrease in my pain when I've paid more attention to being careful about my day-to-day eating.

A November 2021 article by Harvard Health entitled "Foods that Fight Inflammation" included a list of foods that cause inflammation, as well as foods that fight inflammation. In this article, they comment that some foods in a diet that causes inflammation are generally considered bad for our health, including soda, refined carbohydrates, as well as red and processed meats. "Some of the foods that have been associated with an increased risk for chronic diseases such as type 2 diabetes and heart disease are also associated with excess inflammation," Dr. Hu, professor of nutrition and epidemiology at the Harvard School of Public Health states. In an effort to avoid inflammation, try to avoid or limit these foods as much as possible:

- Refined carbohydrates, such as bread and pastas
- French fries and other fried foods
- Soda and other sugar-sweetened beverages
- Red meat (burgers and steaks) and processed meats (hotdogs and sausages)

Dr. Hu goes on to state, "Many experimental studies have shown that components of food or beverages may have an anti-inflammatory effect." Anti-inflammatory foods he lists include:

- Tomatoes
- Olive oil
- Green leafy vegetables like spinach, kale, and collards

- Nuts like almonds and walnuts
- Fatty fish
- Fruits such as strawberries, blueberries, cherries, and oranges

He also lists coffee, which contains polyphenols and other compounds that may protect against inflammation as well. He states that in addition to lowering inflammation, a more natural, less processed diet can have noticeable effects on your physical and emotional health. As I mentioned previously, although I have not followed these suggestions exclusively, I have noticed an improvement, and particularly have sought to reduce or limit those foods listed as inflammatory.

If you suspect that your pain or other symptoms may be due to the effects of inflammation, be sure to consult your doctor or other medical professional to get a second opinion. Everyone is different and it's important to be aware of any food allergies or potential negative interactions with any of your current medications. Also, it's always possible your pain could be from another source other than inflammation.

Improving the Zzzzzs

The other area in which I needed to change my mindset was in regards to sleep. With me personally, I discovered that there were certain vital components

I needed to add to my day in order to predict a better night's sleep:

- Exercise. I realized that personally I am much more likely to sleep well when I feel physically tired. So, for me, my minimum goal is to walk every day. Obviously, the more I do physically, the more tired I am, and the better I sleep. Unfortunately, some days just don't allow for long exercise sessions. When I am seated for longer periods of time, I have found it vital to incorporate a short period of stretching. This can also ward off stiffness and pain.
- Attempt to maintain approximately the same sleeping/waking time schedule. This can be altered slightly, but I have found I am sleeping better as I attempt to wind down between 10:00-11:00 p.m., and get up between 7-8 a.m. This was advice originally given to me by my rheumatologist who diagnosed me with fibromyalgia. This turned out to be good advice.
- Relax my body physically with an Epsom salts bath or a shower, which focuses on tense muscles.
- Relax my mind with soothing music or inspirational reading to take my mind off the cares of the day.

- Relax my spirit. I sleep best when I pray, giving God my cares and worries, and trusting Him to handle the results.
- Some nights I additionally write in a journal, to remind myself of my blessings and answered prayers, giving thanks for the positives of the day.
- Drink a cup of calming herbal tea if for any reason I am not feeling sleepy.
- Be careful to avoid caffeine the second half of the day. Although I have really found coffee and dark chocolate to help my mental focus and concentration, they have been known to inhibit sleep.
- Avoid day sleeping, unless I am really exhausted. A nap can make me less likely to have regular sleep at night.
- If I awaken at night, do my best not to allow myself to get into a "thinking cycle" of trying to solve an issue in the middle of the night. Remind myself that tomorrow is another day, and the issues will still be there in the morning. If necessary, put quiet music back on radio for another ten minutes. Give it back to God in prayer.

In addition to the above tips, I would like to also add one final piece of information, which might go a long way toward benefiting your body with better sleep. I have noticed that numerous times after I've watched television or worked on my computer or iPad late into the evening hours, I tend to struggle with falling quickly into deep sleep. This problem can be directly related to what is termed as "blue light." I have discovered that limiting or even avoiding bright light of any kind can go a long way towards ensuring I more quickly fall asleep.

The reason for this is that researchers have learned that light is linked to your sleep patterns and how it affects your body's natural circadian rhythm. Sometimes also referred to as your "inner clock," your brain cycles through sleepiness and alertness throughout the day at regular intervals. The rising and setting of the sun affects your circadian rhythms based on the amount of sunlight that reaches your eyes. This process also affects your body's production of melatonin, which increases and tends to peak in the middle of the night.

Research has shown that bright light, especially blue light from electronic devices, tends to delay production of melatonin and interrupt sleep patterns. I have personally found that for me, personally, turning off electronic devices and limiting other bright lights around the house for approximately ninety minutes to two hours is most helpful in allowing me to wind down and fall asleep more quickly. If you are unable to do this, you may want to consider the use of blue-light-blocking glasses during the later evening. These glasses have amber lenses that have been shown to block up to 99% of blue light.

I am certain you may come up with additional ideas that may have helped you. If you find in spite of everything, you are not getting adequate sleep, be sure to reach out for help. I would never recommend pretending, as I did, that you can "fake it" until your situation changes. Don't risk injuries or further health issues by denying your body the sleep it really needs! Quality sleep is extremely important for your continued good health and well-being.

I want to encourage you to continue to be a lifetime learner, especially in regards to understanding your own body and brain. Many doctors are overwhelmed with the number of people they are currently helping. They only have so many hours in their days. We can't expect them to always have all the answers regarding our medical issues. For this reason I advise you to do the following things:

- Read online articles and/or books, especially those that give you updated research on your own medical conditions. It may also be helpful if you have not already educated yourself in regards to your condition regarding causes, side effects, and preventative strategies, if applicable.

- Don't be afraid to seek information regarding alternate or alternative treatments for your disorder. For me in particular, I was excited to discover the healing power of stem cells, which I would say has had the greatest impact on my overall condition. I have discovered that many doctors have only been trained in a certain background medically, and may not be aware of everything that's out there that may possibly help you. Again, I want to emphasize the fact that they only have so much available time. I have had the opportunity to share facts with my doctor that he found helpful. Always look at case studies regarding new discoveries, but I will advise you to have adequate information before moving forward. Make new decisions cautiously, after you have carefully done all the necessary research. In my opinion, it may also be a good idea to get multiple opinions, if you are at all in doubt about how you should proceed.

- Be sure you are reaching out to people who are fully trained in their fields, and are also licensed by a governing body.

- Make your overall heath a priority. I urge you, with the advice of your medical team, to make difficult but positive decisions necessary for you to have a happier and healthier tomorrow. Changes may be difficult, but are sometimes necessary.

- Exercise only to your ability, recognizing any medical limitations. Listen to your own body to help aid in preventing injuries. While exercise can benefit so many areas of our body, and also be great for your brain, be careful to increase your repetitions gradually. Take breaks as often as necessary. A licensed professional trainer may be helpful in achieving your goals.

- If you and your doctor decide that making diet changes may be helpful for your overall health, it may be good to integrate changes on a gradual basis. I also suggest that you choose to be under the supervision of a person who is trained and licensed in the field of nutrition who can monitor your progress.

- Do not give up if you are still struggling with your body and/or brain. Be aware that new research is constantly being conducted by major medical institutions. Your breakthrough may be right around the corner!

SECTION TWO

CHAPTER 8

Battling Through Issues with My Mind, Will, and Emotions

While we all, for the most part, have the desire to be positive, happy people, there may come times where our lives are completely out of control. This was descriptive of my situation for a couple of years beginning at the end of 2012, when I was diagnosed with the brain tumor. I will tell you, very thankfully, that my situation definitely improved in the following years. However, for that period of time, life was a real struggle.

This is a difficult section for me to personally write. For close to fifteen years I operated a counseling practice in which I helped many people with their own issues regarding the area of the body sometimes called the "soul," including your mind, will, and emotions. I counseled individuals and couples on many topics for almost twenty years in total. I had earned a PhD in psychology and was an ordained minister in 2002. Then later, in 2012 and into 2013, I was unable to help even myself, let alone anyone else. It was the biggest crisis of my lifetime. I experienced a number of physical issues which drastically affected me emotionally and even spiritually. (The spiritual issues I will cover in section three of this book.) The most difficult hurdles for me to handle after my brain tumor diagnosis were two different issues.

The first one was anxiety after a panic attack in the MRI machine. I seemed to be able to recover from that one-time incident; however, there were after-effects which have caused me to be more fearful than I was in the past. I have to work on managing fearful thoughts. I am not going to spend time on this topic other than to say that there are many types of anxiety. It would take a book to explain them all. I want to reiterate the fact that I am not a medical doctor. It is very important that if you are experiencing anxious thoughts for a period of time that you seek professional help. You need to rule out any biological, physical cause that could be causing your anxiety. Some types of anxiety may benefit from counseling. But, first of all, remember we are three parts—body, soul (mind, will and emotions), and spirit. While I am not attempting to write a section on anxiety, in the following section, I will include information on fear. I definitely had to relearn how to deal with fearful thoughts. I hope you will also find this section helpful.

The next major issue I dealt with post-surgery was depression. I had previously dealt with depression in my midlife years, and depression is common in our family, including my own mother. At that time in my life, my doctor also came to the main conclusion that my depression was primarily due to hormonal changes. Post-surgery, my depression was quite different. I cried every day, feeling hopelessness. In addition, my brain was not able to perform well. I saw zero solutions on the horizon. I believe my depression was the direct result of what I consider to be major "fallout" resulting from my brain surgery.

Like anxiety, depression is an illness that can also originate from biological or physical causes. And like anxiety, there are many categories of depression. All the more reason to make sure there is not a physical cause that needs treatment. Your medical doctor should be able to run lab work to help you to determine if you need medication and if therapy would be advised.

I know from the past, working many years as a therapist, that learning to change your thought patterns may also be very beneficial in dealing with depression. While, again, I am not directly addressing depression due to its very complex nature and treatment, in future chapters I will give you a number of positive tools and suggestions to help you have a more positive mindset. I also will be describing a number of issues that I had to personally battle during the past number of years, and how I personally coped. It is my hope that you may also find these chapters helpful.

CHAPTER 9

Dealing with Fear

As I mentioned earlier, this book is meant to primarily cover injury issues I went through during my illness, ones that others may be also going through at some point in their lives. For me individually, my fear was centered around fear of the future. My biggest fear was that I would not adequately recover, or worse yet, that my life might never be the same. I wanted to again be able to do something to make a difference in other people's lives. As a believer in God, I hate to admit it, but I feared He might not restore my former quality of life. Obviously, those fears, although not ultimately realized, were very real at the time.

Fear is defined as the emotion of alarm in reaction to a perceived danger or threat. The danger may be real—for example, the shadow of a burglar or a rapidly approaching car—or it may be imaginary—for example, a shutter creaking in the breeze, or a scary thing happening in a movie. But the perception is real and defined. What are some common fears that people face? Potential disasters are a big one, such as unemployment, hurricanes, fires, or accidents. Another fear might be simply losing control, which is the fear of becoming vulnerable usually covered up by becoming controlling. What about the fear of being rejected and the fear of being abandoned, which will make a person feel that they're at the mercy of their loved ones? Another fear is simply disappointing people or the need to continually please others to avoid feeling abandoned. Other fears might include things like facing the past, getting trapped or losing an opportunity, or achieving success but still admitting failure. The list goes on and on.

Under this topic of fear, I want to first discuss a common question in our minds when we are fearful, which is "What is going to happen to me?" What are the three common mental mistakes we tend to make?

- We have a tendency to overreact, thinking that a bad thing is going to happen.
- We also tend to further overestimate the consequences of that issue we fear.
- Lastly, we underestimate our ability to cope when the bad thing happens. Also, from my own experience, I think we tend to underestimate the tools and resources that are out there that may be available to help us.

I have had the experience of making all of the above mistakes. In addition, I personally experienced a temporary lack of faith in God for a period of time, which was detrimental to me. I will elaborate more on that in Section Three.

I want to share a few tips that may help you in mastering your fear. First, write down the thought you are having when you experience the emotion of fear. Be honest in confronting your fear by choosing to deal with it. Putting it in writing often helps in this process.

Secondly, be honest with yourself and ask yourself those three questions in the section above. Be honest with yourself over whether you may be overacting, overestimating the issue, or underestimating your abilities or available resources in dealing with your situation. Personally, I've caught myself procrastinating or putting off getting something important done, due to fear of not being able to succeed at completing a task, or finding the help to complete it. That mindset has caused me unnecessary delay and frustration, due to not feeling I was able to move forward with my plans.

For me, it really helps for me to brainstorm and talk with others about my situation. Recently when I did that, the answer more easily came to mind as to how to solve the problem, and I was able to put my fear to rest. I would strongly advise you that if fear is regularly standing in your way of accomplishing your goal, or even just dealing with fears in your life, it might be wise to speak to a counselor, in order to brainstorm your existing fearful feelings. Creating new plans and habits can definitely make your life more hopeful and less stressful in the future. Focus on your abilities and resources that you have at hand. Also, it may help to get more information by reading books on the topic or even articles online. Remember, there are resources out there to help you face your fear.

Lastly, consider using your spiritual side to connect with and put your faith in God. It has been said the opposite of fear is faith. With God all things are possible. As I have personally grown with God spiritually, I have been convinced that God has many times been there to strengthen me, even in my very weakest moments. If I take my focus off of my own fears, and choose instead to focus on how He has ultimately answered so many past prayers, I know I'm never going to give in to living a life of fear. He has always been faithful in getting me through fearful circumstances, when I have chosen to hand my fears over to Him.

CHAPTER 10

Banishing Bitterness

What do most of us people who have bitterness have in common? In my own experience as a counselor and in dealing with my own issues, I believe for most people it's a lack of forgiveness. It's important to know that that lack of forgiveness may be the result of any sort of offense from another person, from yourself, or even God.

What causes bitterness? According to *Psychology Today*, "All bitterness starts as the result of a hurt." We have all felt hurt at times, haven't we? So what's the most important thing concerning that fact? It's really how we handle it. What are some signs or symptoms that you might be bitter (adapted from Aspiringtips.com)?

- In general, you may feel that you have been burned by at least one person in your life, and as a result you've become distrustful of that person, or of people in general.
- You may think that you deserve better than what you've received in the past.
- You may not feel happy about your current life or achievements.

- Because you're feeling generally upset, it takes away from your feelings of happiness.
- You don't always see and appreciate when other people are good to you.
- It may be difficult for you to acknowledge others' skills or even congratulate them for their success.
- You tend to be in general more verbally critical, finding fault in others as your first reaction.
- You may dislike or resent others who are happy, and in turn are negative or display other signs of bitterness.

In addition to the above list, I would also include these signs as well:

- You tend to avoid running into circles of people where you might have a chance meeting with someone you feel has offended you.
- Just the very thought of them results in bad feelings.

By far the biggest downside about retaining bitterness is that it really hurts you individually. One of my biggest challenges in life has been to make the decision to let go of the past and make the choice to forgive. Sometimes it is time to forgive others, or even myself, or in some cases, God. When you're going through a series of very difficult situations individually, I have noticed that there is a tendency to have a negative attitude in general towards everyone, and as a result play the "blame game."

For example, I noticed as I was going through my turmoil of experiencing major sleep loss and pain throughout my body, for some crazy reason I had a tendency to blame other people when it was really no one's fault. I felt let down by the doctors for not finding a solution for my medical condition; this translated into unforgiveness; that turned into bitterness and bad feelings toward them. It was unrealistic, I now realize this, to expect them to have all the answers. Somehow, I think I had also been bitter towards God. I have had to repent for my bad behavior. It is unfair to blame God. Our timing is not God's timing. He has ultimately provided me so much healing in the long run, even if it didn't arrive on my own time schedule. The last person I had to forgive was, believe it or not, myself. As a result of my poor health, I acted out through poor behavior, being negative and critical of others, and only thinking of myself. Also, many times not being emotionally supportive of others. I am being very transparent here, and I have to confess that I'm somewhat embarrassed to admit that these feelings translated into a form of self-hatred. I had changed so much, and as a result, I really had difficulty recognizing the person I had become. I no longer recognized the person I saw in my mirror.

The biggest decision I had to make was the one to forgive all parties, including myself. One thing I have learned through my experiences is that extreme pain issues will bring out the very worst in people. Maybe you know someone who has experienced prolonged pain involving health issues. I'm guessing for the most part they may not be the most cheerful, happy people to be around. I believe that had I not experienced such devastating circumstances with my own health, I would never have fully understood this principle. So, I challenge you: if you're going through something similar, forgive others, forgive God, but most importantly to rid yourself of all the bitterness, forgive yourself. It will bring you unimaginable healing as you rid yourself of all those bad feelings.

These are steps to help you through the process of forgiveness:

1. Make the choice and decision to let go of your bad feelings toward the other person, God, or yourself, and then make the choice to move forward and forgive.
2. Acknowledge your hurt feelings. Include all those instances that have made you upset from

the past regarding each person in which you want to forgive. Take time to write these down on paper. It may also help to talk to someone you trust. Be honest about your feelings, and don't make excuses or apologize for people who have hurt you in the past.

3. Realize that if we are truthful with ourselves, we have all been hurtful or offensive to others during some points of our own lives. If possible, attempt to empathize with the other party. There is no one perfect who has ever walked this earth, other than perhaps Jesus Christ.

4. To completely heal your own heart, be open to praying a prayer to God. In this prayer, ask Him to enable you to forgive this person and also pray for blessings to overtake them. This can be difficult, but shows your true motive, that it is your honest desire to forgive. As you do this, pray for God to heal your own heart.

The above process may need to be repeated for best results. My advice is to make the prayer a regular part of your daily routine. As I have taken the time to make the practice of forgiveness a habit, I have found that not only are there great benefits for me personally, but there is a huge freedom in putting the past to rest. While we can't change what has happened in the past, we can definitely change our reaction to it. Forgiveness doesn't trigger amnesia. Having said that, from my personal experience, praying prayers of blessings over others who have hurt me has been extremely powerful and healing for my own heart.

CHAPTER 11

Getting Through the Difficult Stages of Grief

Sooner or later, we all have to acknowledge the reality of death. Ecclesiastes 3 tells us, "There is a time for everything, and a season for every activity under the heavens: a time to be born and a time to die, a time to plant and a time to uproot, a time to kill and a time to heal, a time to tear down, a time to build, a time to weep and a time to laugh, a time to mourn and a time to dance."

During my illness and recovery, I lost two close friends. Both passed away unexpectedly. Then an even closer friend passed away after many treatments for cancer two years ago. Most recently, in the past few months while working on this book, I lost two more loved ones. I never dreamed that the loss of my eighteen-year-old cat could be so devastating. The last month was so difficult, watching her decline. I am convinced I was already grieving as I wept and deeply mourned her loss, even before her death. Many people I know haven't really understood how devastating it can be to lose an elderly pet who is more like a child, but also a close friend. She was the first thing I saw on my bed when I awoke in the morning. This summer, I grieved for "Happy" for over six weeks.

Then, two weeks ago I also experienced the loss of a close friend who attended our Bible study, and who I had shared a close friendship with for about ten years. Immediately it felt like my grieving had been compounded, as I felt somewhat paralyzed to do anything else but cry. I found it difficult to get out of bed in the morning, let alone do important things that needed to be done. It was then that I realized I personally needed to explore new ways regarding how I might work through my own process of grieving.

One of the very mixed blessings of living to an older age is that, despite the positive fact you have been given the gift of celebrating the privilege of living a longer life, you still have to go through the grieving process as the result of losing many loved ones. I know, after being previously a counselor and therapist, to try to be realistic and not expect my grieving to be over in a couple of weeks. There will be more bouts of sad feelings and more tears to be shed in the process. In time, those will gradually diminish in their intensity and duration. It's just a fact that those individuals we have experienced closer relationships with for longer periods of time will be more difficult for us and take longer to grieve. We need to be patient with ourselves and give ourselves time to work through the difficult process. Ups and downs in our emotions will happen and may come at unexpected times. Personally, I would catch myself just mentioning my loved one's name and the tears would begin to pour uncontrollably. When I attempted to not think about my loss and felt I was "dealing with it," a well-meaning friend would bring it up my loss in a conversation, and I again would break down in tears. There is unfortunately no way to shortcut the time it takes you to grieve the loss of a loved one.

To help you understand grieving better, I am going to list what traditional books say can be involved in the so-called "Four Stages of Grieving" that may lead to recovery (in this particular case, adapting the text from H. Norman Wright's *Recovering From the Losses of Life*). It is important to note, however, that not every person goes through these stages precisely, but that these stages are common for many people.

1. Denial. Denial is a common emotion following a significant loss. It consists of a refusal to accept the loss in an effort to avoid the inevitable pain that will follow.

2. Anger. Anger is when the reality of the loss can no longer be denied, and feelings of unfairness

emerge, giving rise to anger and resentment. This anger may be focused on oneself, on the person or the thing lost, or even on God.

3. Depression. Despair and hopelessness replace anger during this stage and may be accompanied by a lower sense of self-worth and even feelings of guilt. Any emotional adjustments begin to occur here, however, which leads to the fourth stage.

4. Acceptance. At this stage the person begins to see their loss from a true perspective. He or she has discovered ways to tolerate the loss and go on with life.

Help to Recovery

A support group consisting of close friends and/or relatives who can be available to share the grieving is an important source of help on those occasions when the depression becomes overwhelming and too much to handle alone. It personally helped me to talk with close relatives and friends over the phone who simply were "just there" for me during those difficult times.

Large funerals seem to be happening less and less. Families many times prefer to keep the services to including only close family members. In some cases, I see that the family may include others at a celebration of life service which may follow in the months following the funeral. What if you are left to grieving alone? A close friend for over thirty-five years, Trisha, passed away after many cancer treatments and battling extreme illness for a couple of years. Unfortunately, her husband chose no funeral and no celebration of life. Her only son lived on the other side of the country. He was unable to afford the cost of flying home with his wife and large family. So the decision was made by her husband not to conduct any services. I personally feel that this is one of the most difficult situations, not having any mutual friends to share the grieving and no service to attend. I feel blessed that I was able to visit Trisha twice during the year prior to her passing. Although we lived several hundred miles away from each other, we spoke over the phone almost to the very end of her life.

Here are a few other tools for grieving which I personally used that may be helpful for you:

- Looking through old photos help me regain many positive memories of times past.
- Looking at physical memories left behind. For example, Trisha had painted a couple of pictures that she gave me as gifts. Also, I examined small souvenirs I had collected while we took trips together.

- Mainly, I recounted mutual experiences that were exclusively shared only with Trisha. Because she was a friend for so many years, I continue to do this today.
- I spoke with her son in California, who although I had not known personally, felt I already knew him because Trisha had mentioned him so many times. It was a great experience for both of us.
- As I continue to write in a journal, obviously it was cathartic to write about Trisha and look forward to reuniting with her once again in heaven.
- Pray and draw near to God. Ask Him to heal your feelings, and if necessary to fill in the empty space. I personally have found this to be very effective in my own situations.

I want to stress that healthy grieving allows room for old memories and new dreams to exist together. What would that loved one want for you? I think we can say in most cases that our loved ones would want us to continue living our lives to the fullest. If you are struggling with getting through your loss because of unresolved issues or memories, please consider joining a grief support group or speaking with a professional counselor. Unresolved or unfinished grieving can result in some people sinking into a deeper depression. Please remember it's different for everyone, and allow yourself all the time and resources necessary for you to achieve a conclusion to your own personal losses. I also want to mention here that losses that need to be grieved may also include other things; for example, a loss of job or the end of an era, college graduation, or retirement from an occupation. Any change in life circumstances may involve the person going through a period of grieving.

CHAPTER 12

Managing Stress

Stress is defined as physical or emotional tension which can be caused by a variety of physical, chemical, or emotional factors. As we confront new stressful situations, our bodies react physically and emotionally, attempting to return to normal. However, over time this stress, whether good or bad, can create havoc on your body and cause a myriad of problems. WebMD reports that "experiencing stress over the long term, however, can take a real physical and mental toll on your health. Research has shown a connection between stress and chronic problems like high blood pressure, obesity, depression, and more."

When you experience stress on a long-term basis, your brain is exposed to increased levels of the hormone cortisol. This exposure weakens your immune system, making it easier for you to get sick, according to the National Alliance on Mental Illness. They further state that stress can also contribute to worsening symptoms of mental illness, including schizophrenia and bipolar disorder. It is common knowledge that an overload of stress can make everything worse. It is important for you to know what you might be able to improve in your own life to reduce the effects of stress on your body and mind.

When are you most susceptible to stress? People are most vulnerable in these following situations:

- When you don't get enough quality sleep
- When you don't have a network of support around you
- When you experience the death of a loved one
- When you are experiencing a major life change such as moving, starting a new job, having a child, or getting married
- When you are experiencing poor physical health
- Even factors such as not eating well or not caring for your health properly can cause you more stress

Not all stress is bad. Getting rid of all the stress, even positive stress, would make for a boring life for many people. It is important to note here that everyone has his or her own threshold. Certain things that may upset you might not even make one of your friends raise an eyebrow. Some people are affected when they experience large crowds and noisy environments, while others react to silence or having too much free time. We are all different.

For me personally, undergoing unexpected health issues such as being diagnosed with a large brain tumor and then months later with the unexpected diagnosis of fibromyalgia brought me more stress than anything else I had ever experienced. Brain surgery was very stressful, especially not knowing if I would survive. People are surprised when I tell them it was more stressful and difficult dealing with the pain and lack of sleep experienced during fibromyalgia than the nighttime of enduring brain surgery. It lasted much longer in terms of time than my recovery from the brain surgery. As difficult as that whole process of recovery from brain surgery was for me, I could at least see slow progress as far as my improvement in the following months. Dealing with the stress of fibromyalgia was more difficult, as I felt overwhelmed, having no idea if I would ever find a resolution.

As I mentioned earlier, we are all affected differently. What are some physical signs that you may be experiencing stress? Some common signs may include the following:

- Headaches
- Trouble sleeping
- Jaw pain
- Changes in appetite
- Frequent mood swings
- Difficulty concentrating
- Feeling overwhelmed

As I said before, long-term stress can cause cortisol to increase, lowering your immune system and making it easier for you to become ill and experience other problems. As I look at the above list, I realize that I personally experienced five of those seven items during the time I went through physical illness. I look back and wonder how many of these could have been reduced if I had been able to manage my stress better.

Developing a personalized approach to reducing stress can help you manage your mental health condition and improve your quality of life. Once you've learned what your triggers are, experiment with coping strategies. Again, this will be different for everyone. As we go through different experiences in life, in my opinion, we learn from life and may be better able to handle issues in the future. So many times life catches us off guard. It will definitely help us to understand techniques which we personally can apply to our own situations to reduce our own level of stress.

What are some techniques that the National Alliance on Mental Illness recommends? Their online article "Managing Stress" includes the following:

- Accept your needs. Recognize what your triggers are and what situations make you feel physically and mentally agitated. Once you know this, you can avoid them when it's reasonable to do so and to cope when you can't.

- Manage your time. Prioritizing your activities can help you use your time well. Making a day-to-day schedule helps ensure you don't feel overwhelmed by everyday tasks and deadlines.

- Practice relaxation. Deep breathing, meditation, and progressive muscle relaxation are good ways to calm yourself. Taking a break to refocus can have benefits beyond the immediate moment.

- Exercise daily. Schedule time to work outside, bike, or join a dance class. Whatever you do, make sure it's fun. Daily exercising produces stress-relieving hormones in your body and improves your overall physical health.

- Set aside time for yourself. Schedule something that makes you feel good. It might be reading a book, going to the movies, getting a massage, or even just taking time to take your dog on a walk.

- Eat well. Eating unprocessed foods like whole grains, vegetables, and fresh fruit is the foundation for a healthy body and mind. Eating well can also stabilize your mood.

- Get enough sleep. Symptoms of some mental health conditions like mania and bipolar disorder can be triggered by getting too little sleep. (Again,

I want to make a comment here that those of us who had other health conditions that have affected our sleep may need more attention from a physician or even a sleep therapist.)

- Avoid alcohol and drugs. They don't actually reduce stress; in fact, they often make it worse. If you are dealing with substance abuse, educate yourself and get help.

- Talk to someone, whether friends, a family counselor, or a support group. Airing your thoughts by talking can definitely help.

I personally would like to add a few more strategies to this list that have helped me in my own life. I realize adding these make take additional effort, but personally they have paid huge benefits to me:

- Begin your day with a short "quiet time." The length of time will depend on your own availability of time in the morning, but many people have found getting up even ten minutes earlier in the morning to do this results in great benefits, especially in getting your day off to a peaceful beginning. Many times what happens after that is out of my control, but by doing this personally I am able to handle the rest of the day better, because I made this choice. Your quiet time might consist of reading or listening to a short devotional or scripture reading, listening to positive music, or offering up a prayer. Even doing one of these things can be hugely beneficial to getting your day off to a good start.

- If it is at all possible, I recommend repeating the above at the end of the day before retiring. I have especially found it beneficial to relax before bedtime, listening to inspirational music and concluding with prayer, giving God the cares of the day.

- Journaling a paragraph or two in a diary will help remind you of the good things that have happened, keeping your life in perspective. I have done this for a number of years and it has really helped me to count my blessings, even in the midst of negative circumstances.

- If possible, take a little time in your week to volunteer or find a way to give back to others. I have found that this practice definitely helps me be more "other-focused." Although I don't necessarily do this on a weekly basis, I have noticed it definitely benefits others those who do. I know one person in particular who does this on a regular schedule, and he definitely has been become happier and more fulfilled in life. Choose an activity that is of special interest to you.

- If at all possible, consider taking a break from your busy schedule and do a spiritual retreat. While this may take some effort to plan, it can be well worth the effort, and bring you a great rewards personally.

I congratulate you on your desire to make stress reduction a priority in your life. I believe it is well worth the effort and will bring you great benefits to your body and soul. Keep up the good work. Don't forget, every day is a new day and a new opportunity for a new beginning!

CHAPTER 13

Persevering Through Hard Times: Getting Through Life's Difficult Challenges

I am writing this chapter to encourage you, by offering you positive tools and recommendations, to make it through the hard times of life. I would like to give you the glowing report that I was successful in maintaining a positive mindset while going through the complete period of time encompassing my illness and recovery. However, I would be lying. What I will say is that while there were times of despair in which I wanted to give up, thankfully I did not. I believe in my case, much of that reason I was able to persevere had more to do with my faith, which I will share later in this chapter.

Perseverance is defined in the *Oxford English Dictionary* as "persistence in doing something despite difficulty or delay in achieving success." How do you keep on going when the going continues to be very hard? Before I share with you some concrete tools you may find helpful, let me share some quotes on the topic of perseverance with you from some famous people. I hope you will find these quotes to be encouraging.

"If you are going through hell…keep going." —Winston Churchill

"Tough times never last, but tough people do." —Robert Schuller

"Storms make trees take deeper roots." —Dolly Parton

"We have nothing to fear but fear itself." —Franklin D Roosevelt

"The pain you feel today is the strength you feel tomorrow. For every challenge encountered, there is an opportunity for growth." —Unknown

"Every adversity, every failure, and every heartache carries with it the seed of an equivalent or a greater benefit." —Napoleon Hill

"If you feel like giving up, give up on the feeling and give in to the realization that there are endless possibilities waiting to be discovered before you." —Tom Althouse

"Most of the important things in the world have been accomplished by people who kept on trying when there seemed to be no hope at all." —Dale Carnegie

We have a God "who is able to do immeasurably more than we think or imagine, according to his power that is at work within us" (Ephesians 3:20, New International Version).

It's important to remember that you are not alone. There are many people who have and are currently enduring hardships and challenges, and even getting through failures in their lives. There is no one plan which fits everyone. So, where do you begin in the process of moving forward to a better place?

The first step, I believe, is to create a plan or goal. For some of us who have experienced illness, that may simply mean just reaching a point of wellness where we can physically be well enough to create future plans. For others, it may mean to develop a detailed mental road map of what we want to accomplish in the future. If it's possible, I recommend putting your future vision in writing, and setting short- and long-term goals. Do what you are able to do. By that, I mean be realistic regarding where you currently are and where you want to go or what you want to achieve in the future. Also, realize there are going to be long-term goals that may be just that—taking a much longer time to accomplish.

Be realistic and realize there will be setbacks. Obstacles may arise that may delay your goal achievement. Remain calm and attempt to find tools to help you find solutions to problems. Don't be overwhelmed. Remind yourself that for every problem, there is a solution.

Reach out to others to help you. As I mentioned previously, I delayed my own progress because of fear of failure and then procrastinated getting help. By not reaching out immediately to someone who could help me solve the problem, I greatly delayed my progress. Don't be afraid to immediately reach out and request help from others if you find yourself struggling. In my own experience, it may take a few phone calls, but it's well worth your time and effort if it more expediently helps you solve the problems at hand.

Focus on doing your best to make your own self-care a priority. Remember to eat a healthy diet, exercise, and give yourself plenty of breaks as needed. I have found that when I am going through very difficult times, there are days I simply need to take a breather. That may mean taking the day off, not focusing at all on my difficulties that day but doing something completely different, such as taking a long walk, getting a massage, watching a funny movie or doing any other activity that relieves the day's stress.

Remember, persevering is an ongoing process. Resist the desire to quit. According to researcher Angela Duckworth in her 2010 paper on the subject, "All forms of learning and mastery require perseverance." That learning may require more from us also going through the process of getting through very difficult circumstances.

Duckworth argues that perseverance plus passion equals "grit." Passion is understood here as a strong consistency of interest that provides the underlying motivation for reaching long-term goals. In her bestselling 2016 book, *Grit: The Power of Passion and Perseverance*, she shows that grit is an essential for success in life: "Our potential is one thing. What we do with it is quite another." While aptitude, skills, and a basic degree of talent are important determiners of success, they are not as significant as hard work and trying again and again to improve what we do. This reminds me of the old saying, "If at first you don't succeed, try, try again." The most important point being keep trying... don't give up!

I want to give you a few examples of people who have displayed perseverance to achieve their goals. One such person was Thomas Edison. At one point he said,

"I have not failed. I've just found 10,000 ways to make a lightbulb that don't work." But eventually his persistence paid off. Sir Richard Branson was dyslexic and struggled in school. He failed many exams and was considered a problem student. Rather than dwelling on his academic challenges, he focused on his strengths. I personally feel this a huge key in finding what will work for you. By focusing on his strengths, he became one of the most successful businessmen in Great Britain. J.K. Rowling, who was hugely successful as the author of the Harry Potter series, wrote her first manuscript as a single mother who lived on welfare. When she was rejected by numerous agents, she did not give up. As a result, she became hugely successful, and is now one of the richest women in the world.

I also want to add one more. When I was recovering from surgery and really struggling to cope with my situation, my pastor gave me some great advice, which was to read the Psalms. This was very therapeutic for me, as I discovered David also had many struggles with his life. He was fearful of his enemies and even losing his life. Like me, at one point he even believed God had left his presence. Although he had many personal issues which made him a very imperfect person, and he experienced many ups and downs in life, he persevered. At one point, because he persevered, he killed a giant with a single stone and later was described as "a man after God's own heart." If you read the Psalms, you will understand also the love of God and how that love can give people the perseverance to continue, even when times are difficult. Allow me to share with you an excerpt from Psalm 34:18-19: "The Lord is close to the broken-hearted and saves those who are crushed in spirit. The righteous person may have many troubles, but the Lord delivers him from them all." This scripture was a particularly encouraging sign to me that I would eventually get through those difficult times.

Another section of scripture that particularly encouraged me was 2 Corinthians 12:9, which states, "My grace is sufficient for you, for my power is made perfect in weakness." For a number of years, the best word I can use to describe myself was "weak." God definitely provided much strength for me over and over again. When I felt totally incapable of doing alone, under my own resources, He was my source of strength to get through difficult circumstances. I have to give the credit to God. My faith in Him to help me was my biggest key to persevering through life's great trials.

In concluding this chapter, want to share with you some great benefits of persevering through hard times:

- You learn so much from persevering through your own struggles. You in turn have much hope to offer others in helping them also get through their struggles.

- Your confidence increases as a result of conquering many obstacles.
- Your faith in God may also increase, as you make the choice to lean on Him. Very true for me!
- Personally, I feel like I learned new skills necessary to attempt problem-solving.
- From having to persevere through difficult times, it has made me more appreciative of other people who used their time and resources to help me.
- Perseverance has allowed me to develop patience. I now realize the amount of time necessary at times to see positive results. I am more prepared for the future.

I want to wish you the very best, as you press forward in difficult circumstances, to persevere to a better life.

CHAPTER 14

How to Live a More Positive Life While Living in a Negative World

There are a number of articles addressing the topic of positivity if you choose to do your own online research. However, as a psychologist who has actually had to survive living in a negative world while undergoing chronic illness, I think that you will find my perspective quite different. It is one thing to be healthy and to deal with a negative world. However, for those of us who have also had to battle illness or some type of physical recovery, and deal with trying to stay positive, it is a completely different type of challenge. It is my goal in this chapter to offer a number of different recommendations.

As I personally have found these ideas to be personally helpful for many people, please know that not every suggestion may benefit everyone. Everyone is in a different place. Timing is important and sometimes it's necessary to wait for certain changes in your circumstances to make a new decision that may positively impact your future. If you are unsure or feel conflicted,

I recommend that you seek a professional therapist or get a second opinion from another knowledgeable person before making any changes. However, don't fear moving forward. Even making a single change can have a big impact on having a better, more positive future.

With the pandemic affecting so many people these past couple of years, there have been more reports of anxiety and depression than ever before. When you open your news app or newspaper, or even turn on your television, what do you often see? "Bad news" is the answer I so frequently hear people say in response to that question. Many people have already had to deal with health issues themselves, or have lost loved ones, so many find themselves grieving over their losses. So what is the additional response to not wanting to hear more bad news? The response I most frequently hear is, "I don't listen to the news anymore." I am shocked at the large number of people who have given me that similar response. Some people doubt the journalistic objectivity of the news media, but most tell me that just don't want to expose themselves to the general negativity of these broadcasts. People are seeking ways to be happy by making new happier choices for the future. This point brings me to the first point regarding having a more positive life while living in a negative world, which is to choose positivity over negativity.

Make the decision to be wise about what you expose yourself to on radio, television and social media. All of this input from the outside world makes a huge difference in your own thinking, life decisions, and peace of mind. We need to be careful when we automatically believe everything we hear or see. Decide for yourself if and how you are being impacted. Are you feeling more fearful or pessimistic about the future? It is easy to make those overestimations which cause fear to become a problem that we discussed earlier under the "Overcoming Fear" section. Make the right decision for you to have a more positive, happier future.

Make the decision to be more of an optimist and less of a pessimist. Optimism can provide a variety of benefits, including reducing your stress levels, possibly having better mental and physical health, and having a better future outlook. There is a saying that goes, "So a man thinks . . . he is." Our thinking is displayed in our words and actions. It can be difficult to be around someone who is negative or pessimistic all the time. Sometimes it can be a temporary condition caused by life's circumstances, such as chronic illness or another difficult life issue. However, when it persists, if most of us are honest, we would probably say we try to avoid constantly pessimistic people. How can we train our brains to be more optimistic, so we are less likely to become one of those people? I would like to offer a few suggestions.

- Begin your day with positivity. Read a positive devotion or reading material, or listen to positive words using an app or other media source which is focused on positive, helpful information.
- Start you own day by making a list of positive things you want to accomplish to make it a better day.
- Strive for positive interactions with others. Show genuine interest in others, looking for opportunities to give compliments or congratulate them for a job well-done.
- If at all possible, choose positive people with whom to spend your time. Sometimes, for example in work or home situations, this is not always possible. However, whenever you have the choice, do your best to include other people into your world who are also striving to be optimistic.
- Look for the good when difficult situations arise. Be determined to find a solution, as much as you are able, to a challenging issue.
- Challenge any "automatic negative thoughts" that come to your mind. Sometimes old pessimistic

thoughts come back to haunt us. For example, "This is not going to turn out good," or even "This is an impossible situation." Instead, commit yourself to changing your thoughts to positive ones. For example, "There is a solution for every problem," or "The day is not over yet; things can improve as the day goes on."

- Work on purposefully finding and focusing on positive thoughts. We are given this advice from the words of the Apostle Paul in Philippians 4:8 "Fix your minds on what is true, and honorable, and right, and pure, and lovely. Think about things that are excellent and worthy of praise." Zig Ziegler once stated, "Positive thinking will let you do everything better than negative thinking will." Finally, please contemplate this anonymous quote: "Think positive, be positive, and positive things will happen."

- Conclude your day by purposely focusing on all your positive accomplishments, both large and small. Go further to count your blessings and be thankful to God for everything you have been given. Making the effort to put this in writing in a journal will create a habit of celebrating the positives in life.

In addition, I would like to advise you to consciously make positive choices to benefit yourself regarding your ideology or faith and values. By making choices to embrace a system that leads to positive faith and results in a positive mindset, it will reap rewards that will translate into peace with God and others, creating a happier future. (More concerning this topic will be discussed in Section Three of this book.)

Finally, I want to share some very personal strategies I was able to personally implement in my own life to be more positive, many of which were during very negative times when I was experiencing many physical issues and my options were limited:

- Recounting happy memories via photos and videos of joyful life events have added much joy to my life, both now and in the past. Unfortunately, since brain surgery I experience issues with long-term memory. I am convinced that if I didn't record these memories via smartphone, some I would not remember ever happening.
- Adding positive music to my daily schedule has consistently been a huge benefit to making me feel more joy and peace. I rotate styles of music. I like to listen to soft instrumental music as I write. However, when I wake up and

prior to sleeping, I prefer louder, more vocal inspirational music.

- It really helped me when I was stuck at home due to illness to simply call and reconnect with old friends. Revisiting happier times and experiences always seem to give me a positive boost.

- Journaling and incorporating a gratitude list, being grateful to God for the good things, kept me grounded and more positive, in that I had to pay attention to what was going right, not just focus on what was wrong.

- Creating a more positive vibe by repainting my bedroom a happier, more light-reflective color, or even adding a new colorful rug, has helped my mood by giving me a positive change.

- Getting more sunshine, by consciously making a physical move to either sit on the porch or walk when I was able, improved my emotional disposition while giving me a healthy dose of vitamin D.

- Adding colorful fresh flowers, or even bright artificial ones, to my living space seemed to positively brighten my day.

- As I felt better able to entertain, we invited friends over to the house, and had some group get-togethers. Bible studies and small parties with people we love added positivity to our home environment. Personally, I have also enjoyed making new acquaintances with other positive people. New positive friendships can definitely add happiness to your life.

- Attending positive church services, social events, dance events, and exercise classes have all added tremendously to making my life more positive. While these activities may not all be to your liking, I would say it doesn't hurt to try something new. You never know; you might be surprised at the result. You will never know if you don't take a chance.

- Consider giving God a chance be a part of your life, if you are not already doing so. The best part about having a relationship with God is that He always provides unconditional love and acceptance, and best of all provides you strength when at times your "tank is totally out of gas." My life is testimony of this. He was with me through the good, the bad, and the ugly . . . which I will chronicle next in Section Three.

SECTION THREE

Chapter 15

God, Where Are You?

Back in 2012, following my brain surgery and during my long recovery from fibromyalgia, I went through a very up and down "season" regarding my relationship with God. Things in my life began to change in a spiritual sense. Prior to that time, I had had pretty much what most people would consider a calm, content, and fairly predictable relationship with God. I had asked God to come into my life as a young child, been baptized, and at one point rededicated my life to God at a later point in time. During the vast majority of circumstances, from my point of view, I had experienced God's love and interaction my life in very predictable, positive ways. God was my consistent companion.

However, in 2012 things began to change. After I awoke from a nearly eight-hour brain surgery in early December of that year, in addition to experiencing major physical and emotional problems, the unthinkable occurred. I felt a total spiritual void. I cried out, "God, where out you?" I was totally convinced God had mysteriously left me. It is difficult for me to explain this loss, but I was unable to detect His presence in an way, shape, or form. In my emptiness, I felt totally abandoned.

My husband attempted to comfort me by pointing out that others had experienced the same issue. There was an entire book once written on the topic, in fact, entitled *Dark Night of the Soul*. It was written by a Carmelite monk known as John of the Cross. John's advice was that "during a dark night of the soul, people should not try to meditate on theological issues, but rather should allow their souls to be quiet and tranquil." He further said (in Book 1, Chapter 10) that "the purpose of the dark night is to liberate the soul from the stumbling block of human reasoning and to allow the soul to give full attention to God, while appearing to receive nothing in return." Obviously, this is intensely challenging, because it requires a person to apply a strong faith in order to believe God is present, even though He cannot be seen or felt in the darkness. In my case, I felt this was easier said than done.

As chronicled in my previous book, *Supernatural Rescue*, I would love to tell you that my faith was so strong, I never doubted the presence of God in my life even for one moment. Unfortunately this was not the case. As I read the Psalms I realized I was not alone in my doubting. There were times David also doubted God. In Psalm 10:1-2, David cried out, "Why do You stand afar off, O Lord? Why do You hide Yourself in times of trouble?" Then again, it is recorded in Psalm 13:1 that David calls out to God, "How long, Lord? Will you forget me forever? How long will you hide your face from me?" Reading those verses provided a small comfort in knowing that others have also felt the loss of God's presence. I was not alone and having those feelings.

I recently discovered that Mother Teresa, one of the greatest people who has ever lived in my opinion, experienced doubts and struggles in her religious beliefs. She expressed it this way: "Where is my faith? Even deep down there is nothing but emptiness and darkness. If there be God please forgive me. When I try to raise my thoughts to heaven, there is such convicting emptiness that those very thoughts return like sharp knives and hurt my very soul." After ten years of doubt, Mother Teresa described a brief period of renewed faith. She wrote to spiritual confidant, Michael van der Peet, "Jesus has a very special love for you. But as for me, the silence and emptiness is so great, that I look and do not see - listen and do not hear - the tongue moves, (in prayer), but does not speak....I want you to pray for me - that I let Him have a free hand." She clearly knew that God existed, but at that point, she still felt a void of His presence.

Recently, I also read an article online and viewed a video about a current-day missionary who felt abandoned by God. Pastor Andrew Brunson, who had been a missionary to Turkey for over twenty years, was jailed for two years unexpectedly, with no knowledge of any charges for eighteen months. He admits to feeling forsaken at times by God during periods of being isolated, with at times no contact with the outside world. Fortunately he was finally released after two years of imprisonment.

To conclude my story, although I only experienced a short period of abandonment which I have described in my former book as the "Ten Dark Days," these ten days were by far the worst anxiety I had ever felt, and a loss so much greater than anything I had ever experienced in life. Devastated. I felt my pain was lesser but similar to what Christ must have felt when He cried out, "My God, my God, why have you forsaken me?" (Matthew 27:46, Mark 15:34).

It was ten days after the surgery, December 24, when I experienced the darkest of those ten days. I am going to quote from my book *Supernatural Rescue* the exact order of events as to what happened next.

December 24, 2012. It was Christmas Eve and it turned out to be the last and darkest of the 10 dark days. It was at that point that I reached the very depths of hopelessness. I felt no desire to eat or drink, or to do anything else for that matter. I do not remember leaving the living room couch the whole day. Fear encompassed me and I felt powerless to move around. For some strange reason I did not feel I even had the energy to call out to my husband for help, nor did I want to make any effort to go upstairs to locate him. I don't remember him checking on me, but I did not care. I felt I was completely at the end of my rope and that there was no hope at all. With God out of reach, I had no reason to want to live.

As darkness scattered, I begin to wish to see my mother who had passed away the previous year. What happened next, I have difficulty putting into words. It was a surreal experience.

I begin to feel my spirit drift in and out of my body. As it moved further from my body, I felt a strange comfort that the end was at last drawing near and that my suffering would soon be over.

Evening passed into night. I still felt my soul trying to leave my physical body, getting further and further away. It was at a point of going outside the walls going out of my home. I called out, "God, where are you? What did I do to deserve you leaving me?" These thoughts played in my hopeless mind. I felt physically and spiritually empty.

Then suddenly I saw a huge muscular hand come out in front of me, the hand encompassing my drifting spirit and forcefully pulling it back into my physical body. I instantly knew this was the hand of God. He had miraculously rescued me. I spoke to Him out loud. "God, you are finally back."

Still he did not answer me, strangely choosing silence. My mind was filled with many questions that needed answering. Thankful for His rescue, I remained deeply hurt and grieving. What was the meaning of this experience, which seem to be the turning point of this most painful and tragic season of my life?

In the days to come, I remained emotionally fragile, crying daily when I recollected the pain of those dark fearful days where I received no answers. I still felt very alone and I began to develop a fear of God, but it was not a healthy fear. If God could allow this, then what might He allow next? I wondered. And what terrible thing must I have done to make Him desert me? Why, God, why? Why did He allow me to go through this pain and sorrow? I had feelings of anger with Him. In fact, I was so angry with Him that speaking to God in a conversational way was a thing of the past. I turned to repeating the Lord's Prayer religiously in an attempt to normalize my prayers, but I knew in my heart that it was more of a way of keeping God at a distance. The unexplained absence of God's presence for those ten long and dreadful days had devastated me, and my emotional pain was unremitting.

More weeks passed by and day after day I cried out an anger and frustration, "God, why? Why?" I continued to feel damaged both emotionally and spiritually. Having survived a major surgery that had left the frontal lobe of my brain severely affected, I felt God had chosen to abandon me at a time when I needed him most. I believe I went through a period of grieving the loss my former life, when things were more "normal."

I am glad that God could handle my feelings of anger and extreme disappointment. I eventually began to recall how much God had forgiven me in the past, and in time I made the decision to forgive God for not being there when I felt I most needed Him. Although I could not possibly understand why God allowed this abandonment to happen, the scriptures explain: "As the heavens are higher than the earth, so are my ways higher than your ways and my thoughts than your thoughts." (Isaiah 55:9).

There is no way to explain the "whys" of life. I gradually began to finally deal with sorrow and anger, and my time of grieving the temporary loss of His presence finally was concluded.

Eventually, I remember being able to say, "God, I miss our closeness." And at another point I began to have personal conversational prayer with Him again. I realized that having this closeness with Him was more important than staying in a place of anger, and most importantly I realized that God was faithful to me. Or as I put it in *Supernatural Rescue*, "In truth, He had rescued me. The dawn had returned."

CHAPTER 16

God, Why Haven't My Prayers Been Answered?

I was thankful that God had returned and that our relationship was closer to being back to normal. However, in the months following my brain surgery, I discovered that I was now in new territory, having to live with pain issues on a regular basis, and in addition to that not being able to sleep well. When I say not being able to sleep well, I'm talking about some nights not getting any sleep at all. Unfortunately, lack of sleep translated into more pain, and the cycle of pain and sleep issues continued. I believe I shared earlier in the book the adverse effect that fibromyalgia had on my emotions. I became the kind of person that is very difficult to be around, in that lack of sleep brought out the very worst in me. Not only was I short-tempered and impatient with others, I became very impatient and upset with God, and couldn't understand why He was not answering my prayers for physical healing. I began to wonder if I had done something to deserve this physical pain and suffering. I remembered asking my husband, Jim, "What did I do? Why is God punishing me? For many years, I've served God as a nonprofit counselor, doing multiple mission trips and other volunteer work aimed at helping others and as a means of ultimately honoring God with my gifts. So, why am I being punished?" Jim simply told me, "You didn't do anything wrong." But none of it made sense, and I was feeling worse with each passing day.

Due to ongoing physical issues, I was in no way able to return back to my counseling practice. However, when I realized my ninety-eight-year-old father in Ohio needed help, I gladly made the commitment to travel north from my home in Jacksonville, Florida, to see what I could do to be of help to him. He and I had a few of the same issues: issues with falls, memory issues, and head pain. In addition, we both had problems with sleeping well. I made a few trips to Ohio over the next months. I was thankful I could do something to help someone. Since I was unable to run my counseling practice, I had been feeling somewhat useless. Deep down inside, I wondered if would ever recover from the sleep/pain issues and get my former life back. I was still questioning God. Why can't I get totally well? What have I done that You don't want to heal me?

On one of those trips to Ohio, I had what I would call a major meltdown. In the process of trying to help Dad with a minor repair, I experienced a painful electrical shock while in the kitchen area that, simply speaking, "put me over the edge." I went out into the garage and cried, "God, why didn't You allow me to die?" I was referring to previous times when I had the brain surgery or during the ten dark days when I felt myself slipping away. I was so tired and weary, physically exhausted and tired of being in pain. I was angry at God for allowing it all to continue.

However, I am so glad that He could handle it and wasn't angry in return. I knew He still loved me. You may ask me, "How could you be so sure at that point in time?" I am going to share this excerpt regarding my experience from my book, *Supernatural Rescue*. After retiring for the night at my normal time, the events of that night were not the normal.

At roughly 3 AM I woke but I thought I was dreaming. I could see a bright, deep-looking sky with blue color streaming from the middle of the ceiling. It was alarming to the point I felt my body jump. Was it a bad dream? I was taken aback in fear. I wanted to slap myself awake to escape whatever was happening in my sleep. Then suddenly I realized this was not a dream and that I was fully awake. As I looked into the glaring blue light, I realized that there was a figure present, a body of sorts in the center of the light. As I watched, it was apparent that the figure was watching me. Then very slowly the figure moved away. It was not until the next morning that I realized that I'd seen an angel from God which He had sent to let me know that I was not alone in my pain and suffering. It was exactly what I needed after the previous night's events. This was the first time that I'd ever seen an angel. It was an incredible blessing and I knelt down and thanked God.

After this experience I immediately knew in my soul that the purpose of this holy visitation was to give me hope for the future. Although the prior day I questioned my right to yell out to God in anger, I now have come to understand that I believe God wants us to communicate honestly with Him, whether it means we are happy, sad or angry. Since that time, I have reminded people that it's okay to cry out to God in anger. He knows your heart anyway, and just wants you to reach out to Him in an honest way. No, I wasn't instantly healed at that moment. However, I felt He had responded to my pain and given me a sign, signifying that He heard me call out to Him, and that there was hope for a better future down the road.

I think I have come to understand that there are a number of reasons why we are not having our prayers immediately answered. On this particular occasion, I felt the message was, "Not now, but have hope for the future." There was an unknown reason, but I needed to be patient and wait.

Isaiah gave words of comfort to His people in Isaiah 40. However, he didn't immediately answer their prayers, but told them they would have to wait a while. These are the words of Isaiah: "But those who wait on the Lord shall renew their strength. They shall mount up with wings like eagles. They shall run and not be weary. They shall walk and not be faint" (Isaiah 40:31, New King James Version).

While we wait, we must remember God is still with us. We are not alone in the process. And He promises us strength to get through our dilemmas. Many times, we don't know why we are waiting. There may be many different reasons that only God knows. What we want now might not be in God's timing. By this, I mean that situations may need to happen or events need to fall into place. Other times, God may be doing a "work" inside of us that takes a process of time to be concluded. Romans 5 may help us understand this principle better: "We can rejoice to when we run into problems and trials, where we know that they help us develop endurance. And endurance develop strength of character, and character strengthens our confident hope of salvation. And this hope will not lead to disappointment. For we know how dearly God loves us, because he's given us the Holy Spirit to fill our hearts with his love" (Romans 5:3–5, New Living Translation).

I must say, I have not always been at a place where I can honestly say that I was rejoicing in my problems and trials. However, I will say that in the long-term that may now be true, as I've now been able to share my story through all the problems to get to the "other side." I believe that having to go through years of pain and suffering may encourage others and give them hope that they can also reach a point of peace with their own situations. I think both my situations had to change, and I personally also had to change, in order to get a place of "celebration." There was definitely a waiting period.

What are other reasons our prayers don't get answered? Sometimes we may have wrong motives or lack of faith, or even sometimes God has a different plan. Sometimes God says, "No . . . at least for this period of time." In the New Testament, we are told Paul was given a "thorn in the flesh." Scholars argue as to what that actually means. But what we do know is that Paul begged to God to "take it away" three different times, and the scripture shows no record of that happening (2 Corinthians 12:7–8, NKJV).

God's answer came in the following verse: "My strength is made perfect in weakness" (2 Corinthians 12:9). The New International Version puts it this way: "And he said to me my grace is sufficient for you, for my power is made perfect in weakness. Therefore I will boast all the more gladly about my weaknesses, so that Christ power may rest in me" (2 Corinthians 12:9).

2 Corinthians 12:9 has become what I describe as a new "life verse" for me. The reason I tell you this is that although I have received a measure of "healing," there still exists a number of physical problems which may never be healed, due to having a major brain surgery and resulting fibromyalgia. It's not that I don't have faith that they might be resolved. I know that with God, all things are possible. Having said that, living in weakness has made me even more aware of and dependent on God's faithfulness and strength! Thank you, God, for being there for me through illness, pain, and lack of sleep these past ten years, allowing me to accomplish more than what I would have dreamed could be possible. I am so glad that we serve a God who can do "immeasurably more than we than we ask or imagine, according to his power that is at work within us" (Ephesians 3:20).

CHAPTER 17

God, Do You Still Love Me?

I don't know if you have ever asked God the above question. I hate to admit this truth, but there have been times when I questioned God's love for me.

As I shared with you earlier, I was impatient and upset with God for not immediately answering prayers. I was angry when He "allowed" difficult circumstances, and when I couldn't perceive His presence. I also questioned if God was punishing me for any bad behavior, and that somehow I was deserving of God's "payback." Because of these negative feelings, at times there were brief moments that I questioned His love.

As you examine your own relationship with God, maybe you have also experienced brief time periods where you questioned if God loves you. For some of us, it may come from life circumstances, but for others it may come from perceived failures in your personal life or possibly feeling that you are unable to live up to God's standards. Maybe you failed another person close to you, or have what you perceive as unforgivable sins. Or it could be you can't forgive God for allowing something bad to happen that was out of your control, so you have "cut him off." For these or other reasons, you may have felt an absence of God's love, at least for a period of time.

After I recovered from the most major parts of my illness, I personally had to go back and reacquaint and revisit what I had previously known about God's love. In spite of all that had happened to me, it was most encouraging that God Himself had not changed. It was more about me. My circumstances at times made me see Him differently, but thankfully for only a temporary time period.

One of the first things I needed to remind myself of was that although my thoughts and feelings may change from day to day, we are told God's love does not change. For us, as human beings, it's important for us to realize that sometimes our thoughts and feelings are incorrect, or at least partially false or even based on incomplete information. I know for me personally, those feelings toward God were greatly affected by my negative circumstances.

I want to share with you some information you may not know regarding God's great love for you and me.

God created us "in his own image" (Genesis 1:27).

He "knit us together in our mother's womb" (Psalm 139:13).

His thoughts toward us "outnumber the sand on the seashore" (Psalm 139:18).

God "rejoices over you with singing" (Zephaniah 3:17).

Gods future for you has been "filled with hope" (Jeremiah 29:11).

God is "close to the broken-hearted . . . and those crushed in spirit" (Proverbs 34:18).

He is "the Father who comforts us in all our trouble, so that we may comfort others" (2 Corinthians 1:4).

One day, "He will take away all our pain, and wipe away every tear from our eyes" (Revelation 2:34).

This is such great news for all of us going through difficult times. He still loves us, no matter what happens, regardless of our feelings about Him during life's circumstances.

What about if you feel you have also drawn away from God, by in some way "disconnecting" yourself or purposefully pulling away? How do you attempt to reconnect or get back in relationship with Him? Deuteronomy 4:29 tells us that we will seek Him and find Him, when we seek Him with all our heart and all our soul. What does this mean? I think if I'm honest, in the past I may have only searched for Him half-heartedly. I firmly believe that this may require us to be more purposeful in seeking God, and to continue to seek Him on a more regular schedule. I have found that the more time I invest in what I call my "God" time, the closer I feel to God in our relationship.

If you desire to connect or reconnect with God, my first step would be to speak to God in prayer and tell Him that you want Him in your life. If you have already done that, you might consider a prayer to Him that you want to re-commit your life. I have done this several times in my life, when I felt my relationship with Him had slipped down my list of priorities. Make it a new daily priority to spend time with God. I have discovered the more I do this, the more personal peace I experience. I have tried to make it a priority to have regular prayer times, also devotional and/or reading of scripture to keep myself closer to Him. In addition, I like to jot down a paragraph or two at the end of the day, thanking Him for the day's blessings. As I tend to have memory issues, this can be a great encouragement to go back and re-read these at a later date. Fellowship with other believers can also strengthen our commitment to God. We have found special joy as we prayer for each other, and then share later how those prayers were answered.

What if you are still struggling with your past as far as previous issues? This may involve having to forgive others and also accept God's forgiveness. The great news is God never expects us to be perfect people. Two of the greatest characters in the Bible were both murderers at one point in their lives, David and Paul. David, who committed murder, at one point in the Old Testament was described as "a man after God's own heart." Paul, after murdering countless Christians, became one of the greatest apostles of the New Testament.

It seems pretty certain to me that God is a God of mercy and grace, who doesn't hold our past against us. Know that God did everything necessary to cover your past. God sent Jesus to die and be the propitiation for our past wrongs. We just have to accept God's free gift to us. So what do we need to do next? Simply be honest and admit your past mistakes to God. There is no one perfect. Put our faith in Christ. He has promised to take our "sins as far away as the east is to the west." The scripture says "If we confess our sins, He is faithful and just to forgive us our sins, and cleanse us from all unrighteousness" (1 John 1:9 NKJV). Then, trust God that He's "got your back." The great news is when we become believers, we are promised the gift of the Holy Spirit, who continues to abide with us and be that "still small voice" to offer us wisdom. In addition, Romans tells us that "Spirit helps us in our weakness, and intercedes for us, in accordance with God's will"

(Romans 5:26–27). We will never be alone if we ask God to walk beside us.

The great news is that every day is a new day to set new goals for our lives. If we fall back in any way, God is still there. The great news is we now have a new identity. The old is washed away. All is new.

These are some of the additional blessings we now can also claim as followers of Christ, according to scripture.

I am a joint heir with Christ, sharing His inheritance with Him. (Romans 8:17)

I am a new creation. (2 Corinthians 5:17)

I am a temple, a dwelling place, of God. His Spirit dwells in me. (1 Corinthians 3:16, 6:19)

I am a fellow citizen with the rest of God's family. (Ephesians 2:19)

I am chosen of God, holy and dearly loved. (Colossians 3:12, 1 Thessalonians 1:4)

We know that in all things God works for the good of those who love him, who have been called according to his purpose. (Romans 8:28)

Our future home is heaven. Jesus tells us in John 14:1, "Do not let your heart be troubled. Trust in God's, trust also in me. In my Father's house, there are many rooms. I go there to prepare a place for you . . . that where I am . . . you may be also." He further described heaven the thief who was crucified next to him on the cross as "Paradise" (Luke 23:43 NIV). Psalms 16:11 also advises us that God will "fill us with joy in your presence, with eternal pleasures at your right hand." We have much to look forward to . . . as we look to our future with God in heaven!

I would like to use this final moment of my book to further confirm God's great love for you as His new creation. "If God is for us, who can be against us? He who did not spare his own Son, but gave him up for us all - how will he not also, along with him, graciously give us all things? Who will bring any charge against those whom God has chosen? It is God who justifies. Who is he that condemns? Christ Jesus, who died - more than that, who was raised to life - is at the right hand of God and is also interceding for us. Who shall separate us from the love of Christ? Shall trouble or hardship or persecution or famine or nakedness or danger or sword? No, in all these things we are more than conquerors through him who loved us" (Romans 8:31-35; 37). "For I am convinced that neither death nor life, neither angels nor demons, neither the present nor the future, nor any powers, neither height nor depth, nor anything else in all creation, will be able to separate us from the love of God, that is in Christ Jesus our Lord" (Romans 8:31–39 NIV).

Thanks be to God for His great declaration of love for us! Let us in return show appreciation to God by living a life which aims to give Him all our honor and praise, in all we say and do.

For Further Reading

Harvard Health Newsletter. Go online to health.harvard. edu.

Exercisecoach.com gives you scientific support for the general benefits of exercise and strength training.

"Benefits of Social Dancing." *New England Journal of Medicine*, September 1, 2016.

"Benefits of Brain Boosting Foods." *Medical News Today*, June 27, 2019.

International Society for Cell and Gene Therapy, "Stem Cell Based Therapy for Human Diseases." *Nature*, August 2022.

"Eating for Inflammation." *WebMD*. Retrieved from their website summer 2022.

Dr. Frank Hu, "Foods that Fight Inflammation." *Harvard Health Newsletter*, November 16, 2021.

"Nine Mental Habits That Can Make You Feel Bitter." *Psychology Today*, September 18, 2019.

Norman Wright, *Recovery from the Losses of Life*. Revell Publishing, 2019.

"Stress." *WebMD*. Retrieved from their website summer 2022.

"Managing Stress." National Alliance on Mental Illness website, August 10, 2014.

Angela Duckworth, *Grit: The Power and Passion of Perseverance*. Scribner, 2016.

St. John of the Cross, "Dark Night of the Soul." Circa 1578–1585, now in the public domain.